FOOD LIST
FOR THE
MIND DIET

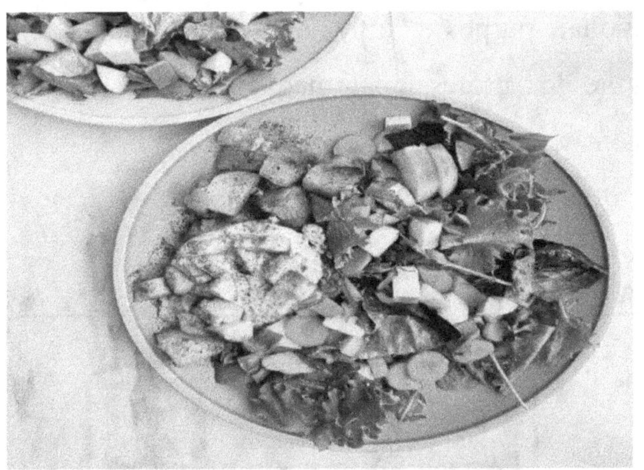

"A Complete Guide and Recipes to Enhance Brain Health, Prevent Dementia, and Alzheimer's"

Dayna G. Murphy

Copyright © 2024 by Dayna G. Murphy

All rights reserved.

Disclaimer: The information provided in this book is for educational purposes only and is not intended as a substitute for professional medical advice, diagnosis, or treatment.

GAIN ACCESS TO OTHER BOOKS BY ME

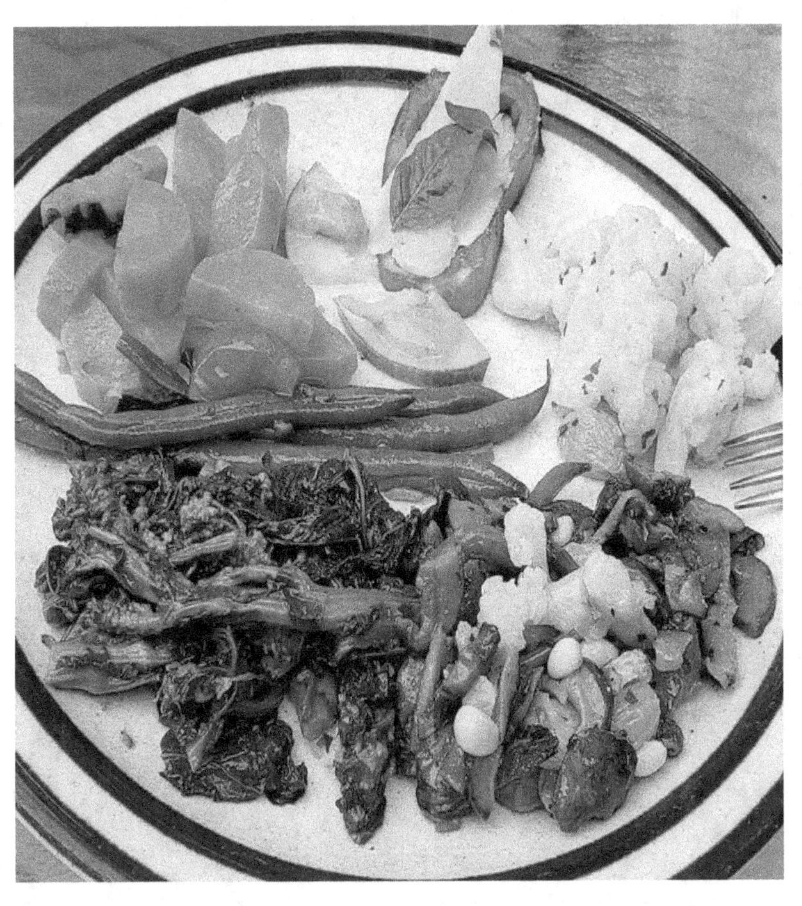

TABLE OF CONTENTS

INTRODUCTION

In the quiet corridors of our minds, the echoes of our daily choices resonate, shaping the very fabric of our mental well-being. Imagine a scenario where a simple adjustment to your daily diet becomes the key to unlocking hidden reserves of mental clarity and vitality. Picture a moment where the fork you lift holds not just sustenance for your body but a secret elixir for your mind.

Meet Jenna, a busy professional navigating the demanding realms of a career that seemed to pull at the edges of her sanity. Amid deadlines and obligations, Jenna stumbled upon a revelation that changed the trajectory of her mental landscape. It wasn't a groundbreaking discovery in a scientific lab or a revolutionary pharmaceutical breakthrough. No, it was a shift in what she chose to put on her plate.

In the pursuit of peak cognitive performance, Jenna embraced the principles of the Mind Diet – a fascinating exploration into the intersection of nutrition and mental well-being. Little did she know that this journey into mindful nourishment would not only fortify her brain against the daily onslaught of stress but would also illuminate a path to sustained focus, emotional resilience, and a profound sense of clarity.

As we embark on this culinary odyssey through the corridors of the Mind Diet, you, too, will uncover the tales of individuals like Jenna whose lives were irrevocably altered by the choices they made at mealtime. Join us as we unravel the science, savor the flavors, and discover the extraordinary impact of food on the extraordinary machine that is your mind. The journey begins with a fork, a plate, and the promise that what you eat has the power to shape not just your body, but the very essence of your cognitive existence."

Purpose of the Book

"In the pages of 'Mindful Nourishment: A Comprehensive Guide to the Food List for the Mind Diet,' our mission is clear — to empower you with the knowledge and tools needed to harness the transformative potential of the Mind Diet. This book is not just a collection of recipes or nutritional advice; it is a roadmap to optimize your cognitive function and elevate your mental well-being. By delving into the intricacies of mindful nutrition, backed by scientific insights, we aim to guide you towards a lifestyle that not only nourishes your body but enriches your mind. Join us on this journey, where the right food choices become a source of vitality, clarity, and sustained mental health. Let the power of mindful nourishment unlock your fullest cognitive potential."

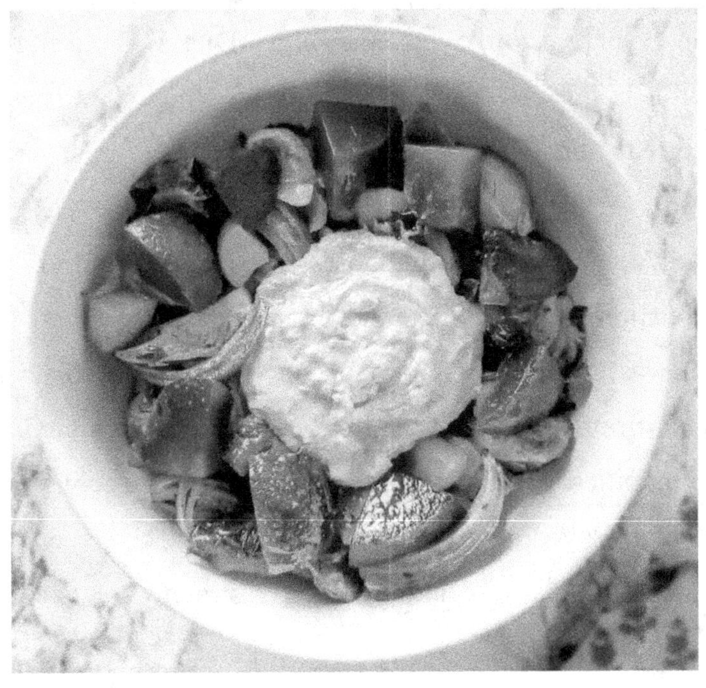

CHAPTER 1: UNDERSTANDING THE MIND DIET

Introduction to Mind Diet

The Mind Diet, short for "Mediterranean-DASH Diet Intervention for Neurodegenerative Delay," isn't just a regimen; it's a culinary symphony designed to harmonize with the intricacies of the human brain. Rooted in a fusion of the Mediterranean and DASH (Dietary Approaches to Stop Hypertension) diets, the Mind Diet is a nutritional approach tailored not only to satisfy the palate but to nurture the brain.

Originating from groundbreaking research on the correlation between diet and cognitive health, the Mind Diet was crafted with a singular objective – to shield the mind from the wear and tear of time. Inspired by communities where age-related cognitive decline was notably delayed, researchers sought to distill the essence of these dietary patterns into a cohesive strategy for fostering brain resilience.

In our exploration of the Mind Diet, we unravel the culinary secrets of cultures where dementia and cognitive decline are rare guests. From the sun-drenched coasts of the Mediterranean, where olive oil flows like liquid gold, to the heart-healthy strategies of DASH, this dietary amalgamation transcends mere nourishment, offering a blueprint for a vibrant and mentally resilient life.

Scientific Basis

At the heart of the Mind Diet lies a profound understanding of how specific nutrients function as allies in the battle for cognitive well-being. The science behind this dietary paradigm is a tapestry woven with intricate threads of neurology, biochemistry, and nutrition.

1. Omega-3 Fatty Acids:

- Dive into the role of omega-3s, the brain's preferred fatty acids, in enhancing synaptic function and mitigating inflammation.

2. Antioxidants:

- Explore the antioxidant-rich foods that stand sentinel against oxidative stress, protecting delicate brain cells from premature aging.

3. Vitamins and Minerals:

- Unpack the significance of vitamins such as B-complex and minerals like magnesium and zinc, pivotal in neurotransmitter synthesis and overall cognitive function.

4. Polyphenols:

- Examine the vibrant world of polyphenols found in fruits, vegetables, and tea, and their potential to combat cognitive decline through anti-inflammatory and antioxidant mechanisms.

CHAPTER 2: THE POWER OF MINDFUL EATING

Mindful Eating Practices:

In a world where meals are often hurried affairs and multitasking is the norm, the concept of mindful eating emerges as a sanctuary for our mental health. Mindful eating is not just a technique; it's a transformative approach to nourishing both body and mind. It invites us to savor the symphony of flavors, textures, and aromas that dance on our plates, anchoring us in the present moment.

1. Present Moment Awareness:

- Delve into the essence of mindful eating, where each bite becomes a conscious experience. Explore the practice of being fully present, free from the distractions that often accompany mealtime.

2. Engaging the Senses:

- Uncover the sensory richness of food. From the vibrant colors to the satisfying crunch, mindful eating encourages us to engage all our senses, forging a deeper connection with the act of nourishment.

3. Non-Judgmental Observation:

- Embrace a non-judgmental stance towards food. Mindful eating encourages us to observe our thoughts and feelings without criticism, fostering a healthier relationship with what we eat.

4. Recognizing Hunger and Fullness:

- Explore the intuitive wisdom of the body. Mindful eating teaches us to recognize hunger and fullness cues, empowering us to respond to our body's needs with attunement.

Benefits of Mindful Eating:

The ripple effects of mindful eating extend far beyond the dinner table, touching the very core of our cognitive well-being. As we cultivate a mindful approach to nourishment, a cascade of benefits unfolds, each contributing to the resilience and vitality of our minds.

1. Stress Reduction:

- Uncover how mindful eating acts as a powerful antidote to stress. By grounding us in the present moment, it becomes a meditative practice, alleviating the mental burdens that often accompany our fast-paced lives.

2. Enhanced Focus and Concentration:

- Explore the correlation between mindful eating and improved cognitive function. By fostering a heightened awareness, this practice becomes a catalyst for enhanced focus and concentration.

3. Emotional Regulation:

- Delve into the emotional intelligence that arises from mindful eating. By tuning into our emotions during meals, we develop a mindful response to stressors, contributing to emotional resilience.

4. Healthy Relationship with Food:

- Discuss how mindful eating nurtures a positive and balanced relationship with food. As individuals become attuned to their body's signals, they develop a sustainable and nourishing approach to eating.

CHAPTER 3: MIND DIET FOODS LIST

MIND DIET BEVERAGES

1. Water:

- Stay hydrated with pure, filtered water. It's essential for overall health, including brain function.

2. Green Tea:

- Rich in antioxidants and beneficial compounds, green tea has been associated with cognitive benefits.

3. Coffee:

- Moderate coffee consumption has been linked to a reduced risk of neurodegenerative diseases. Opt for black coffee or with minimal added sugar.

4. Herbal Teas:

- Teas like chamomile, peppermint, or hibiscus can be enjoyable alternatives without caffeine.

5. Blueberry Juice:

- Blueberries are known for their brain-boosting properties. Enjoying a small glass of unsweetened blueberry juice can be a flavorful option.

6. Pomegranate Juice:

- Pomegranates are rich in antioxidants, and consuming unsweetened pomegranate juice can be a tasty addition.

Recommended Weekly Intake (in milligrams) for Different Age Groups:

Seniors (65+ years):

- **Water:** 7,000 – 10,000 ml per week (approximately 1,000 – 1,500 ml per day)
- **Green Tea:** 14 – 21 cups per week (2 – 3 cups per day)
- **Coffee:** 7 – 14 cups per week (1 – 2 cups per day)

- Herbal Teas, Blueberry Juice, Pomegranate Juice: Enjoy in moderation, keeping added sugars minimal.

Normal Age People (25-64 years):

- **Water:** 7,000 – 10,000 ml per week (approximately 1,000 – 1,500 ml per day)
- **Green Tea:** 14 – 21 cups per week (2 – 3 cups per day)
- **Coffee:** 7 – 14 cups per week (1 – 2 cups per day)
- Herbal Teas, Blueberry Juice, Pomegranate Juice: Enjoy in moderation, keeping added sugars minimal.

Children (4-11 years):

- **Water:** 4,000 – 7,000 ml per week (approximately 600 – 1,000 ml per day)
- **Herbal Teas:** 1 – 2 cups per week (occasional)
- **Fruit Juices:** Limit intake due to added sugars; focus on whole fruits.

Teenagers (12-18 years):

- **Water:** 5,000 – 8,000 ml per week (approximately 700 – 1,200 ml per day)
- **Green Tea, Herbal Teas:** 7 – 14 cups per week (1 – 2 cups per day)
- **Coffee:** If consumed, limit to 7 cups per week with minimal added sugars.
- **Fruit Juices:** Limit intake due to added sugars; focus on whole fruits.

Men and Women (19-64 years):
- **Water:** 7,000 – 10,000 ml per week (approximately 1,000 – 1,500 ml per day)
- **Green Tea:** 14 – 21 cups per week (2 – 3 cups per day)
- **Coffee:** 7 – 14 cups per week (1 – 2 cups per day)
- Herbal Teas, Blueberry Juice, Pomegranate Juice: Enjoy in moderation, keeping added sugars minimal.

MIND DIET FRUITS:

1. Blueberries:

- Packed with antioxidants, blueberries have been linked to improved cognitive function.

2. Strawberries:

- Rich in vitamin C and other antioxidants, strawberries contribute to overall brain health.

3. Blackberries:

- High in anthocyanins, blackberries offer neuroprotective benefits.

4. Raspberries:

- A good source of fiber and antioxidants, raspberries support brain health.

5. Apples:

- Provide dietary fiber and polyphenols, contributing to heart and brain health.

6. Pears:

- Contain fiber and antioxidants, supporting digestive and cognitive health.

7. Oranges:

- Rich in vitamin C, oranges contribute to overall immunity and brain function.

8. Bananas:

- Provide potassium and other essential nutrients important for brain health.

9. Avocado:

- While technically a fruit, avocados are rich in healthy fats and support brain function.

10. Grapes:

- Contain resveratrol, an antioxidant associated with cognitive benefits.

Recommended Weekly Intake (in grams) for Different Age Groups:

Seniors (65+ years):

- **Blueberries:** 150 - 200g per week (1/2 - 3/4 cup, 2 - 3 times per week)
- **Other Fruits:** 500 - 750g per week (1.5 - 2.5 cups per day)

Normal Age People (25-64 years):

- **Blueberries:** 150 - 200g per week (1/2 - 3/4 cup, 2 - 3 times per week)
- **Other Fruits:** 500 - 750g per week (1.5 - 2.5 cups per day)

Children (4-11 years):

- **Blueberries:** 50 - 100g per week (1/4 - 1/2 cup, 1 - 2 times per week)
- **Other Fruits:** 400 - 600g per week (1 - 2 cups per day)

Teenagers (12-18 years):

- **Blueberries:** 100 - 150g per week (1/3 - 1/2 cup, 1 - 2 times per week)
- **Other Fruits:** 500 - 700g per week (1.5 - 2 cups per day)

Men and Women (19-64 years):

- **Blueberries:** 150 - 200g per week (1/2 - 3/4 cup, 2 - 3 times per week)
- **Other Fruits:** 500 - 750g per week (1.5 - 2.5 cups per day)

MIND DIET VEGETABLES:

1. Leafy Greens:

- Kale, spinach, collard greens – rich in folate and antioxidants.

2. Broccoli:

- High in vitamin K and choline, supporting brain health.

3. Carrots:

- Packed with beta-carotene, carrots contribute to overall eye and brain health.

4. Sweet Potatoes:

- Rich in vitamins A and C, sweet potatoes offer neuroprotective benefits.

5. Bell Peppers:

- High in vitamin C and antioxidants, bell peppers support immune function.

6. Tomatoes:

- Contain lycopene, associated with cognitive benefits.

7. Brussels Sprouts:

- Rich in fiber, vitamins, and antioxidants, Brussels sprouts contribute to overall health.

8. Cauliflower:

- A versatile vegetable with compounds linked to cognitive health.

9. Eggplant:

- Contains anthocyanins, contributing to brain health.

10. Onions:

- Rich in quercetin, onions offer anti-inflammatory and antioxidant benefits.

Recommended Weekly Intake (in grams) for Different Age Groups:

Seniors (65+ years):

- **Leafy Greens:** 400 - 600g per week (2 - 3 cups, 4 - 5 times per week)
- **Other Vegetables:** 600 - 800g per week (2 - 3 cups per day)

Normal Age People (25-64 years):

- **Leafy Greens:** 400 - 600g per week (2 - 3 cups, 4 - 5 times per week)
- **Other Vegetables:** 600 - 800g per week (2 - 3 cups per day)

Children (4-11 years):

- **Leafy Greens:** 200 - 400g per week (1 - 2 cups, 2 - 3 times per week)
- **Other Vegetables:** 400 - 600g per week (1 - 2 cups per day)

Teenagers (12-18 years):

- **Leafy Greens:** 300 - 500g per week (1.5 - 2 cups, 3 - 4 times per week)

- **Other Vegetables:** 500 - 700g per week (1.5 - 2 cups per day)

Men and Women (19-64 years):

- **Leafy Greens:** 400 - 600g per week (2 - 3 cups, 4 - 5 times per week)
- **Other Vegetables:** 600 - 800g per week (2 - 3 cups per day)

MIND DIET WHOLE GRAINS:

1. Quinoa:

- A complete protein source, rich in fiber and various nutrients.

2. Brown Rice:

- High in fiber and contains beneficial antioxidants.

3. Barley:

- Packed with fiber, vitamins, and minerals, supporting heart health.

4. Oats:

- Rich in beta-glucans, oats contribute to heart health.

5. Whole Wheat:

- Contains fiber and essential nutrients, promoting overall health.

6. Buckwheat:

- A gluten-free whole grain with antioxidant properties.

7. Farro:

- High in fiber, protein, and various nutrients.

Recommended Weekly Intake of Whole Grains (in grams) for Different Age Groups:

Seniors (65+ years):

- **Whole Grains:** 350 - 500g per week (50 - 70g per day)

Normal Age People (25-64 years):

- **Whole Grains:** 350 - 500g per week (50 - 70g per day)

Children (4-11 years):

- **Whole Grains:** 150 - 250g per week (20 - 35g per day)

Teenagers (12-18 years):

- **Whole Grains:** 250 - 350g per week (35 - 50g per day)

Men and Women (19-64 years):

- **Whole Grains:** 350 - 500g per week (50 - 70g per day)

MIND DIET LEGUMES:

1. Lentils:

- High in protein, fiber, and various essential nutrients.

2. Chickpeas:

- A good source of protein, fiber, and folate.

3. Black Beans:

- Rich in antioxidants, fiber, and protein.

4. Kidney Beans:

- High in fiber, potassium, and iron.

5. Edamame:

- Young soybeans with protein, fiber, and essential nutrients.

Recommended Weekly Intake of Legumes (in grams) for Different Age Groups:

Seniors (65+ years):

- **Legumes:** 250 - 350g per week (35 - 50g per day)

Normal Age People (25-64 years):

- **Legumes:** 250 - 350g per week (35 - 50g per day)

Children (4-11 years):

- **Legumes:** 100 - 200g per week (15 - 30g per day)

Teenagers (12-18 years):

- **Legumes:** 150 - 250g per week (20 - 35g per day)

Men and Women (19-64 years):

- **Legumes:** 250 - 350g per week (35 - 50g per day)

MIND DIET FISH:

1. Salmon:

- Rich in omega-3 fatty acids, particularly EPA and DHA.

2. Mackerel:

- High in omega-3s and other essential nutrients.

3. Sardines:

- A good source of omega-3s, calcium, and vitamin D.

4. Trout:

- Contains omega-3 fatty acids and is a good protein source.

5. Tuna:

- Especially valuable if fresh or canned in water, providing omega-3s.

Recommended Weekly Intake of Fish (in grams) for Different Age Groups:

Seniors (65+ years):

- **Fish:** 250 - 350g per week (2 - 3 servings per week)

Normal Age People (25-64 years):

- **Fish:** 250 - 350g per week (2 - 3 servings per week)

Children (4-11 years):

- **Fish:** 150 - 200g per week (1 - 2 servings per week)

Teenagers (12-18 years):

- **Fish:** 200 - 300g per week (2 - 3 servings per week)

Men and Women (19-64 years):

- **Fish:** 250 - 350g per week (2 - 3 servings per week)

MIND DIET POULTRY:

1. Chicken Breast:

- Lean source of protein, low in saturated fat.

2. Turkey:

- Lean meat, a good source of protein and other nutrients.

3. Quail:

- A lean poultry option, providing protein and various vitamins.

Recommended Weekly Intake of Poultry (in grams) for Different Age Groups:

Seniors (65+ years):

- **Poultry:** 350 - 500g per week (2 - 3 servings per week)

Normal Age People (25-64 years):

- **Poultry:** 350 - 500g per week (2 - 3 servings per week)

Children (4-11 years):

- **Poultry:** 150 - 250g per week (1 - 2 servings per week)

Teenagers (12-18 years):

- **Poultry:** 200 - 300g per week (2 - 3 servings per week)

Men and Women (19-64 years):

- **Poultry:** 350 - 500g per week (2 - 3 servings per week)

MIND DIET OILS AND FATS:

1. Olive Oil:

- Rich in monounsaturated fats and antioxidants, beneficial for heart and brain health.

2. Canola Oil:

- A good source of omega-3 fatty acids and low in saturated fat.

3. Avocado:

Contains monounsaturated fats, fiber, and various vitamins.

4. Nuts and Seeds:

- Almonds, walnuts, flaxseeds, and chia seeds are rich in omega-3 fatty acids, fiber, and antioxidants.

5. Fatty Fish:

- Salmon, mackerel, and sardines are excellent sources of omega-3 fatty acids.

Recommended Weekly Intake of Oils and Fats (in grams) for Different Age Groups:

Seniors (65+ years):

- **Healthy Oils and Fats:** 350 - 500g per week (2 - 3 servings per day)

Normal Age People (25-64 years):

- **Healthy Oils and Fats:** 350 - 500g per week (2 - 3 servings per day)

Children (4-11 years):

- **Healthy Oils and Fats:** 150 - 200g per week (1 - 2 servings per day)

Teenagers (12-18 years):

- **Healthy Oils and Fats:** 200 - 300g per week (2 - 3 servings per day)

Men and Women (19-64 years):

- **Healthy Oils and Fats:** 350 - 500g per week (2 - 3 servings per day)

Tips for Healthy Fats and Oils Intake:

1. Use Olive Oil for Cooking:

- Incorporate extra virgin olive oil in cooking and salad dressings.

2. Include Avocado in Meals:

- Add sliced avocado to salads, sandwiches, or as a topping.

3. Snack on Nuts and Seeds:

- Include a handful of nuts and seeds as a snack or sprinkle them on yogurt or salads.

4. Choose Fatty Fish:

- Include fatty fish like salmon, mackerel, or sardines in your diet regularly.

5. Limit Saturated and Trans Fats:

- Reduce intake of foods high in saturated and trans fats, such as processed and fried foods.

MIND DIET DAIRY:

1. Greek Yogurt:

- High in protein and probiotics, supporting gut health.

2. Milk (preferably low-fat or skim):

- A good source of calcium and vitamin D for bone health.

3. Cheese (preferably low-fat):

- Provides calcium and protein, but moderation is key due to higher fat content.

4. Cottage Cheese:

- A protein-rich dairy option with lower fat content.

Recommended Weekly Intake of Dairy (in grams or servings) for Different Age Groups:

Seniors (65+ years):

- **Dairy:** 700 - 1,000g per week (3 - 4 servings per day)

Normal Age People (25-64 years):

- **Dairy:** 700 - 1,000g per week (3 - 4 servings per day)

Children (4-11 years):

- **Dairy:** 500 - 700g per week (2 - 3 servings per day)

Teenagers (12-18 years):

- **Dairy:** 700 - 900g per week (3 - 4 servings per day)

Men and Women (19-64 years):

- **Dairy:** 700 - 1,000g per week (3 - 4 servings per day)

Mind Diet Eggs:

Eggs:

- Excellent source of high-quality protein and essential nutrients, including choline.

Recommended Weekly Intake of Eggs for Different Age Groups:

Seniors (65+ years):

- **Eggs:** 4 - 7 eggs per week (1 egg every other day)

Normal Age People (25-64 years):

- **Eggs:** 4 - 7 eggs per week (1 egg every other day)

Children (4-11 years):

- **Eggs:** 3 - 5 eggs per week (1 egg every 1-2 days)

Teenagers (12-18 years):

- Eggs: 4 - 7 eggs per week (1 egg every other day)

Men and Women (19-64 years):

- **Eggs:** 4 - 7 eggs per week (1 egg every other day)

Tips for Incorporating Dairy and Eggs:

1. Include Yogurt in Breakfast:

- Add Greek yogurt to your breakfast with fruits or nuts.

2. Choose Low-Fat Dairy:

- Opt for low-fat or skim milk and cheese to reduce saturated fat intake.

3. Enjoy Eggs in Various Forms:

- Include eggs in your diet through omelets, boiled eggs, or as an ingredient in meals.

4. Use Dairy in Cooking:

- Use dairy products in cooking and baking to enhance nutrient intake.

5. Monitor Portion Sizes:

- Be mindful of portion sizes, especially for higher-fat dairy options.

MIND DIET NUTS:

1. Almonds:

- Rich in monounsaturated fats, vitamin E, and magnesium.

2. Walnuts:

- High in omega-3 fatty acids, antioxidants, and polyunsaturated fats.

3. Pistachios:

- A good source of protein, fiber, and various vitamins and minerals.

4. Cashews:

- Provide healthy fats, iron, and zinc.

5. Brazil Nuts:

- High in selenium, a powerful antioxidant.

Recommended Weekly Intake of Nuts (in grams) for Different Age Groups:

Seniors (65+ years):

- **Nuts:** 150 - 200g per week (1/2 - 3/4 cup, 2 - 3 servings per week)

Normal Age People (25-64 years):

- **Nuts:** 150 - 200g per week (1/2 - 3/4 cup, 2 - 3 servings per week)

Children (4-11 years):

- **Nuts:** 75 - 100g per week (1/4 - 1/3 cup, 1 - 2 servings per week)

Teenagers (12-18 years):

- **Nuts:** 100 - 150g per week (1/3 - 1/2 cup, 2 - 3 servings per week)

Men and Women (19-64 years):

- **Nuts:** 150 - 200g per week (1/2 - 3/4 cup, 2 - 3 servings per week)

MIND DIET SEEDS:

1. Flaxseeds:

- Rich in omega-3 fatty acids, fiber, and lignans.

2. Chia Seeds:

- High in fiber, omega-3 fatty acids, and various nutrients.

3. Pumpkin Seeds:

- A good source of magnesium, iron, and zinc.

4. Sunflower Seeds:

- Contain vitamin E, magnesium, and selenium.

Recommended Weekly Intake of Seeds (in grams) for Different Age Groups:

Seniors (65+ years):

- **Seeds:** 75 - 100g per week (1/4 - 1/3 cup, 2 - 3 servings per week)

Normal Age People (25-64 years):

- **Seeds:** 75 - 100g per week (1/4 - 1/3 cup, 2 - 3 servings per week)

Children (4-11 years):

- **Seeds:** 50 - 75g per week (2 - 3 tablespoons, 1 - 2 servings per week)

Teenagers (12-18 years):

- **Seeds:** 75 - 100g per week (1/4 - 1/3 cup, 2 - 3 servings per week)

Men and Women (19-64 years):

- **Seeds:** 75 - 100g per week (1/4 - 1/3 cup, 2 - 3 servings per week)

Tips for Incorporating Nuts and Seeds:

1. Snack on Mixed Nuts:

- Create a mixed nut snack with a variety of nuts.

2. Sprinkle Seeds on Meals:

- Sprinkle seeds on salads, yogurt, or smoothie bowls.

3. Include Nuts in Breakfast:

- Add nuts to your breakfast, such as oatmeal or yogurt.

4. Use Nut Butters:

- Choose natural nut butters for spreads or as ingredients in recipes.

5. Incorporate Seeds in Baking:

- Use seeds in baking or as toppings for muffins and bread.

CHAPTER 4: FOODS TO LIMIT OR AVOID

The Mind Diet encourages a focus on nutrient-rich foods that are beneficial for brain health. To optimize cognitive function and reduce the risk of neurodegenerative diseases, it's advisable to limit or avoid certain foods that may contribute to inflammation, oxidative stress, and other factors linked to cognitive decline. Here are some general guidelines on foods to avoid or limit in the Mind Diet:

Foods to Limit or Avoid:

1. Red and Processed Meats:

- High intake of red and processed meats has been associated with an increased risk of cognitive decline. Limit the consumption of beef, pork, and processed meats like sausages and bacon.

2. Butter and Margarine:

- High levels of saturated fats found in butter and some margarines may contribute to cardiovascular issues, which can affect brain health. Choose healthier fat sources like olive oil.

3. Cheese and Full-Fat Dairy:

- While dairy is included in the Mind Diet, it's recommended to choose low-fat or fat-free options. High-fat dairy products may contribute to increased saturated fat intake.

4. Fried and Fast Foods:

- Foods deep-fried in unhealthy oils and fast food items often contain trans fats and excessive amounts of unhealthy fats. These may contribute to inflammation and cardiovascular issues.

5. Sweets and Sugary Snacks:

- High sugar intake has been linked to cognitive decline. Limit sugary snacks, candies, and desserts. Opt for natural sweeteners in moderation.

6. Highly Processed Foods:

- Processed foods often contain additives, preservatives, and unhealthy fats. Minimize the intake of pre-packaged, processed foods, and focus on whole, minimally processed options.

7. Sodas and Sugary Drinks:

- Sugary beverages can lead to insulin resistance and have been associated with cognitive decline. Choose water, herbal teas, and unsweetened beverages instead.

8. Excessive Alcohol:

- While moderate alcohol consumption may have some benefits, excessive drinking can harm the brain. If you choose to consume alcohol, do so in moderation.

9. Highly Salted Foods:

- High sodium intake may contribute to hypertension, affecting brain health. Limit the consumption of highly salted and processed foods.

10. Artificial Additives and Preservatives:

- Some studies suggest a potential link between artificial additives and preservatives and cognitive decline. Opt for natural, whole foods whenever possible.

General Tips:

1. Moderation is Key:

- Enjoying a balanced and varied diet is crucial. Moderation in all food choices is a key principle of the Mind Diet.

2. Stay Hydrated:

- Proper hydration is essential for overall health, including brain function. Choose water as the primary beverage.

3. Individual Considerations:

- Factors such as allergies, sensitivities, and individual health conditions should be taken into account. If in doubt, consult with a healthcare professional or a registered dietitian for personalized advice.

CHAPTER 5: MIND DIET MEAL PLANS AND RECIPES

Sample Meal Plans:

Day 1:

Breakfast:

- Greek Yogurt Parfait with Mixed Berries and a Drizzle of Honey
- Whole Grain Toast with Avocado

Lunch:

- Grilled Salmon Salad with Leafy Greens, Cherry Tomatoes, and Olive Oil Dressing
- Quinoa on the side

Snack:

- Handful of Almonds and Walnuts

Dinner:

- Baked Chicken Breast with Lemon and Herbs
- Roasted Vegetables (Broccoli, Carrots, Brussels Sprouts)
- Brown Rice

Day 2:

Breakfast:

- Oatmeal with Chia Seeds, Banana Slices, and a Sprinkle of Nuts
- Green Tea

Lunch:

- Whole Wheat Wrap with Turkey, Hummus, Spinach, and Tomatoes
- Mixed Veggie Sticks on the side

Snack:

- Greek Yogurt with a Spoonful of Flaxseeds

Dinner:

- Quinoa-Stuffed Bell Peppers with Lean Ground Turkey
- Steamed Asparagus
- Mashed Sweet Potatoes

Recipes:

Avocado and Berry Smoothie:

- **Ingredients:** 1/2 avocado, 1/2 cup mixed berries, 1 banana, 1 cup spinach, 1 cup almond milk.

- Blend all ingredients until smooth. Optional: Add a scoop of protein powder for an extra boost.

Mediterranean Salmon Salad:

- **Ingredients:** Grilled salmon, mixed greens, cherry tomatoes, cucumber, red onion, Kalamata olives, feta cheese, olive oil dressing.
- Toss all salad ingredients together and drizzle with olive oil dressing.

Quinoa-Stuffed Bell Peppers:

- **Ingredients:** Quinoa, lean ground turkey, bell peppers, black beans, corn, tomatoes, onion, garlic, cumin, paprika.
- Cook quinoa and sauté turkey with vegetables and spices. Stuff bell peppers with the mixture and bake until peppers are tender.

Meal Prep Tips:

1. Batch Cooking:

- Prepare grains (quinoa, brown rice) and proteins (chicken, salmon) in bulk at the beginning of the week to use in various meals.

2. Chop and Store Veggies:

- Wash, chop, and store vegetables in the fridge for easy access. They can be added to salads, wraps, or stir-fries throughout the week.

3. Make-ahead Smoothie Packs:

- Portion out smoothie ingredients into bags or containers and freeze. In the morning, simply blend with liquid for a quick and nutritious breakfast.

4. Prep Snack Packs:

- Create snack packs with a mix of nuts, seeds, and dried fruits. These are convenient and healthy options for on-the-go snacking.

5. Freeze Individual Portions:

- Freeze individual portions of soups, stews, or casseroles for quick and easy microwave meals when time is limited.

6. Build-a-Bowl Concept:

- Create a "bowl" with a base (quinoa, brown rice), a protein (chicken, beans), and a variety of veggies. Make several combinations for diverse meals.

7. Pre-cut Fruits:

- Wash, slice, and store fruits like berries, melons, and citrus in the fridge for easy access during the week.

8. Use Mason Jars for Salads:

- Layer salads in mason jars, starting with dressing at the bottom and adding greens and toppings. Seal and refrigerate until ready to eat.

Meal prepping can save time, ensure you have nutritious options readily available, and make it easier to stick to the

Mind Diet principles. Adjust portion sizes and ingredients based on individual needs and preferences.

CONCLUSION

In the conclusion of "Nourish Your Mind: A Mind Diet Guide," we reflect on the transformative journey toward optimal cognitive well-being. The Mind Diet, a holistic approach to nourishing both body and mind, has equipped us with the knowledge to make intentional food choices that positively impact our mental health. As we've explored the rich tapestry of nutrient-dense foods, delving into the vibrant world of fruits, vegetables, whole grains, lean proteins, and healthy fats, we've discovered the power of culinary choices in fortifying the brain against the challenges of aging.

This book aimed not just to provide information but to inspire a lifelong commitment to mindful eating, fostering cognitive resilience and enhancing overall vitality. The scientific foundations, delectable recipes, and practical meal plans offer a roadmap for integrating Mind Diet principles into our daily lives. The importance of moderation, diversity, and conscious food choices resonates as we recognize that nourishing our minds goes beyond a single meal—it's a lifestyle.

As we bid farewell to these pages, let us carry the wisdom gained within our culinary endeavors, savoring each bite as an investment in the longevity and vitality of our most precious asset—the mind. May every meal be a celebration of health, a symphony of flavors that harmonize with the intricate dance of neurons. Embracing the Mind Diet is not just a dietary choice; it's a declaration of self-care, an ode to a life well-lived, mindfully and deliciously.